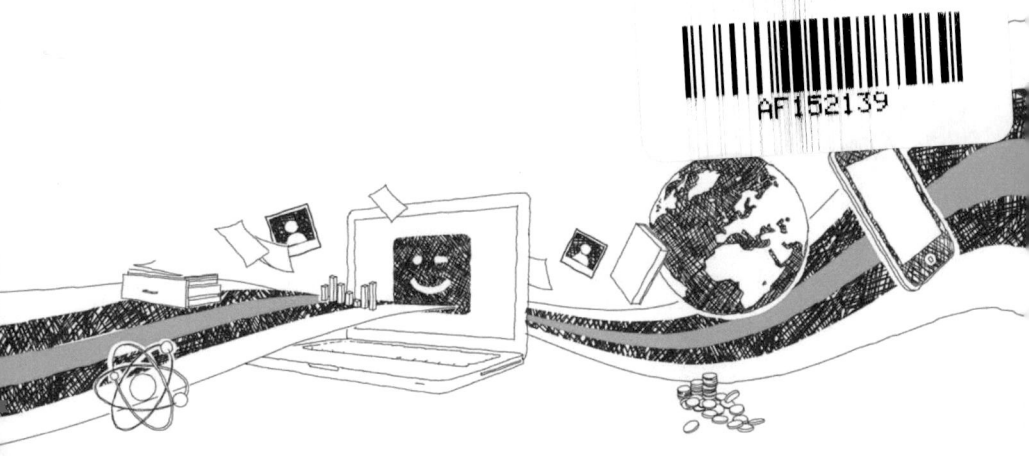
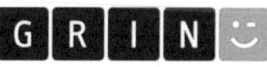

Carol Nganga

Soy Foods and Isoflavones: Cause or Inhibit Breast Cancer?

GRIN Publishing

Bibliographic information published by the German National Library:

The German National Library lists this publication in the National Bibliography;
detailed bibliographic data are available on the Internet at http://dnb.dnb.de .

Imprint:

Copyright © 2011 GRIN Verlag GmbH
Print and binding: Books on Demand GmbH, Norderstedt Germany
ISBN: 978-3-656-73936-4

This book at GRIN:

http://www.grin.com/en/e-book/280533/soy-foods-and-isoflavones-cause-or-inhibit-
breast-cancer

GRIN - Your knowledge has value

Since its foundation in 1998, GRIN has specialized in publishing academic texts by students, college teachers and other academics as e-book and printed book. The website www.grin.com is an ideal platform for presenting term papers, final papers, scientific essays, dissertations and specialist books.

Visit us on the internet:

http://www.grin.com/

http://www.facebook.com/grincom

http://www.twitter.com/grin_com

Does the Consumption of Soy Foods and Isoflavones in Particular, Cause or Inhibit Breast Cancer?

Introduction

The impact of soy foods on potential breast cancer risk has been a topic of considerable investigation in the medical field. The primary importance of research on soy foods is derived from the fact that these foods are rich in isoflavones, which are supposedly associated with inhibition of breast cancer development (Messina & Wood, 2008, p.1). Isoflavones are mainly contained in soybeans. High soy food intake in Asian countries like Japan is said to have sparked research on the role of isoflavones on reduction of breast cancer in 1990s (Messina & Wu, 2009, p.1673). Some isoflavones such as genistein possess non-hormonal properties that are associated with breast cancer inhibition in women. Thus, it is highly prudent to say that there are several mechanisms by which soy may reduce the risk of breast cancer in women. However, recent epidemiological studies have provided evidence suggesting that isoflavones indeed promote breast cancer (Kang *et al*, 2010, p.1859). This is because isoflavones such as geinstein have been found to stimulate growth of breast cancer cells which are estrogen-sensitive in overectomized mice. Several *in vitro* studies have shown that isoflavones can both inhibit or enhance ability of drugs to fight breast cancer (Nagata, 2010, p.83). Thus, understanding of the effects of isoflavones on breast cancer is still vague. This paper explores whether consumption of soy foods and isoflavones cause or inhibit breast cancer in women. In section 1, definitions of Isoflavones, biological functions and endocrine therapies will be given. In section 2, supporting literature on the positive and negative effects of isoflavones will be discussed. In section 3, several studies will be used as examples to support the information provided in section 2.

Hypothesis

If women consume soy foods high in isoflavones, they will reduce their risk of breast cancer.

Research question

The research question for this study was; "is it important for women to understand the benefits and risks associated with a diet containing soy foods?"

Justification

Efficacy of isoflavones has persistently been put under scrutiny, and patients have equally become confused on whether or not to consume soy foods (Nagata, 2010, p.83). Therefore, careful evaluation of the available evidence is a viable endevor. It is immensely important to identify the strengths and limitations of this alternative therapy of breast cancer. Therapeutic research has generated the need for statistical design and evaluation. As such, research on breast cancer treatments and therapies has been assigned an important role in the medical field and is seen as a means of reducing dependence conventional treatments (Messina & Wood, 2008, p.2). This research provides adequate information about the efficacy of isoflavones as a potential remedy for breast cancer in the world.

Section 1: Definition of isoflavones, biological effects and relative risk

Isoflavones are diphenolic compounds that are chemically similar to estrogens. Thus, they are elements of phytoestrogens. Phytoestrogens are plant-derived compounds that have biological properties of estrogens (Messina & Wood, 2008, p.2). As such, isoflavones can bind to alpha and beta estrogen receptors. There are three main types of isoflavones; genistein, daidzein and glycitein (Messina & Wood, 2008, p.2). Biological effects of isoflavones can be defined as the various actions which are activated by these diphenolic compounds. Some of these biological actions include: inhibition of cell development, enhancement of cell differentiation, stimulating apoptosis and cell proliferation (Nagata, 2010, p.83).

Tamoxifen and anastrozole, as used in this article, are the commonly used adjuvant endocrine therapies for patients with breast cancer (Kang *et al*, 2010, p.1857). However, they are mostly used for patients who have hormone-sensitive cancer. Relative risk of a disease can be defined as the risk of the disease relative to exposure to various factors. Thus, it is a ratio of probabilities for two distinct factions. Understanding the underlying effects of the isoflavones is important in order to assess efficacy of soy foods in inhibition of promotion of breast cancer. Biological effects of genistein and daidzein should therefore be evaluated.

Section 2: Supporting literature on effects of Soy food on breast cancer

Genistein, which is an isoflavone, is associated with various biological actions which reduce risks of breast cancer. According to Trock, Hilakivi-Clarke and Clarke (2006, p.460), genistein slows down the epidermal development of tyrosine kinase, which is associated with growth of mammary tumors (Nagata, 2010, p.83). In addition, this isoflavone inhibits the activity of topoisomerase II, therefore reducing risks for breast cancer, especially among postmenopausal women (Trock, Hilakivi-Clarke and Clarke, 2006, p.460). However, these anticancer effects occur only at specific experimental conditions.

For instance, inhibition of angiogenesis by isoflavone occurs only when genistein intake is adjusted to pharmacologic concentrations (30-185 µM) (Trock, Hilakivi-Clarke and Clarke, 2006, p.460). Thus, reliance on dietary exposures may not be effective in inhibiting breast cancer growth. Isoflavone intake can also inhibit growth of mammary tumors through modification of various types of metabolism, such as eicosanoid activity which affects cell differentiation (Trock, Hilakivi-Clarke and Clarke, 2006, p.460). This modification process is achieved by restricting cell cycle progression in the body. Thus, it can be deduced that soy food intake reduces risks of breast cancer among women.

2 meta-analyses that were performed on studies involving Asian and Western populations have showed an inverse relation between breast cancer and isoflavone exists (Nagata, 2010, p.83). One of the meta-analysis was based on 8 studies, and it found that soy food intake reduces breast cancer by approximately 29% (Nagata, 2010, p.83). According to Nagata, one of the meta-analysis that was performed on Asian women found out that consumption of more than 20 mg of isoflavones per day can reduce breast cancer by approximately 50%, based on the pharmacologic concentrations (Nagata, 2010, p.83).

According to Nagata (2010, p.84), reduction in growth of breast cancer cells can only be achieved if soy intake is started at an early stage of life. For instance, it is reported that soy intake in Japan starts early in life, a factor that explains the low incidence rates for cancer in Japan (Nagata, 2010, p.84). 32 out of 100,000 women in Japan suffer from breast cancer. In Hawaii, U.S, the incidence rate is estimated to be 107.5 per 100,000 (Nagata, 2010, p.84). This massive difference explains the importance of isoflavone consumption and reduction in breast cancer. Japan's Food Safety Commission has cited that most Japanese families consume 26 to 54 mg of isoflavones each day, hence the low incidence rates of breast cancer among Japanese women (Nagata, 2010, p.84).

Daidzein is an isoflavone which is also effective in reducing breast cancer. This compound is said to enhance the efficacy of cancer treatments such as tamoxifen (Trock, Hilakivi-Clarke & Clarke, 2006, p.469). Apart from their effectiveness in enhancing tamoxifen ability, daidzein in soy foods is also capable of increasing tumor latency, which reduces the growth of cancerous cells in the mammary tissues. Thus, consumption of isoflavones can significantly reduce development of breast cancer in women.

According to Nagata (2010, p.83), isoflavones such as daidzein inhibit the conversion of androgens to estrogens by various enzymes. In addition, these compounds are anti-proliferative and proapoptic. These biological actions are vital in the inhibition of cancerous cell growth in the mammary tissues (Nagata, 2010, p.85). As a result, it can be construed that consumption of soy foods can effectively control growth of breast cancer among women.

Despite the widespread notion that isoflavones reduce cancer risks, several clinical and epidemiological studies have shown otherwise. According to Trock, Hilakivi-Clarke and Clarke (2006, p.460), some properties demonstrated by isoflavones could indeed increase the risk for breast cancer. For instance, some of isoflavones' estrogenic properties could be promoters of breast cancer in women (Nagata, 2010, p.84). Activation of the alpha estrogen receptor is one of such effects which are associated with increased incidence rate for breast cancer.

According to Messina and Wood (2008, p.2), genistein facilitates the proliferation of xenografts which are elements of breast cancer in human beings. In overectomized mice, clinical investigations have found that isoflavones inhibit the action of anti-estrogens such as tamoxifen in cancerous cells that grow as xenografts (Trock, Hilakivi-Clarke & Clarke, 2006, p.469). These characteristics are thus suggestive of possible risk factors for breast cancer. Therefore, it can be deduced that consumption of soy beans causes breast cancer in women.

According to Messina and Wu (2009, p.1675), mice which are implanted with estrogen receptor-positive breast cancer (MCF-7) can portray an increased tumor growth if subjected to high levels of genistein (Messina & Wu, 2009, p.1675). This evidence shows that there is a direct relationship between increase of breast cancer and soy consumption. This stimulation of tumor growth, however, occurs under certain experimental conditions. For instance, tumor growth increases in mice with MCF-7 if estrogen pellets are removed from these rodents (Messina & Wu, 2009, p.1675).

Apart from genistein, daidzein is also associated with increased breast cancer risk if the animals are implanted with estrogen receptor-positive breast cancer. However, most of these studies have not identified any relationship between soy isoflavone intake and breast tissue density (Messina & Wu, 2009, p.1675). Controversies surrounding consumption of isoflavones and growth in breast cancer seem to be unrelenting. Therefore, evaluating several epidemiological and clinical studies can give some insight on relevance of isoflavones.

Section 3: Analysis and findings based on various studies

Many epidemiological studies have shown that breast cancer can be reduced by high intake of soy foods. A prospective study involving respondents from Singapore showed that high intake of soy foods can reduce breast cancer among postmenopausal women by approximately 18% (Wu *et al*, 2008, p.196). In this prospective study conducted on Singapore Chinese women, 35,303 individuals were used as study subjects. The subjects were administered with questionnaires covering 165 food and beverages (Wu *et al*, 2008, p.196).

Using the Cox Regression model, this prospective study generated a relative risk (RR) of 0.82 at 95% confidence interval (Wu *et al*, 2008, p.197). Women who had consumed more than median levels of soy foods (>10.6 mg 1000Kcal^{-1}) experienced 18% reduction of breast cancer risk (P-value= 0.019). However, soy intake was found to be statistically insignificant among premenopausal women, with P-value of 0.08 at 5% percent (Wu *et al*, 2008, p.197). This study therefore shows that soy food intake reduces the risks of breast cancer among women.

Table 1.Soy intake and breast cancer risk, based on the Singapore prospective study

Soy isoflavone (mg 1000 kcal^{-1})	Number of cases	Person-years	RR[a]	95% CI
All subjects				
< 10.6 mg	339	167 312	1.00	
≥ 10.6 mg	290	170 930	0.82	0.70 – 0.97
P-value				0.019
Menopausal status at baseline				
Premenopausal				
< 10.6 mg	84	43 668	1.00	
≥ 10.6 mg	106	52 937	1.04	0.77 – 1.40
P-value				0.82
Postmenopausal				
< 10.6 mg	255	123 608	1.00	
> 10.6 mg	184	117 960	0.74	0.61 – 0.90
P-value				0.003

Source: British Journal of Cancer (2008, p.197)

Concentrations of plasma genistein in the human body were recently found to have implications on breast cancer. A recent cohort study of 24,226 women conducted at the Japan Public Health Center found out that genistein plasma concentrations affect incidence rates of breast cancer (Messina & Wu, 2009, p.1674). The plasma and serum concentration in isoflavones is a factor that affects incidence of breast cancer among women. The protective role played by isoflavones is largely associated with suppression of estrogen receptor-positive cancer tumors (Messina & Wu, 2009, p.1675).

In this study, respondents with higher plasma genistein concentrations had a 30% reduced risk for breast cancer when compared to other respondents. In this study, the p-value was 0.02 at 95% confidence interval. This means that plasma genistein concentrations affect incidence rates for breast cancer (Messina & Wu, 2009, p.1675). This Japanese cohort study was also consistent with a Chinese case-control study that found an inverse relationship between plasma genistein concentrations and breast cancer (Messina & Wu, 2009, p.1675). Thus, it can be construed that soy foods can reduce the incidence rate for breast cancer.

A study conducted between 2002 and 2003 on participants undergoing endotherapy treatment showed that consumption of isoflavones reduces recurrence rates (Kang *et al*, 2010, p.1860). In this study, 524 participants were used. These participants had previously undergone surgery at the Harbin Medical University Hospital in China. The follow-up was done until 2008, after which the study attributes were analyzed using the Cox Regression model (Kang *et al*, 2010, p.1858). The premenopausal women were provided with tamoxifen therapy, whereas postmenopausal participants were undergoing anastrozole treatment as adjuvant endocrine therapy. Their isoflavone consumption was monitored during the follow-ups.

In the four consumption quartiles, the mean intake levels were 6.5, 18.2, 35.8 and 49.6 mg/day respectively (Kang *et al*, 2010, p.1860). After analysis, women in the highest quartile reported reduced cancer recurrence rates than women found in the lowest quartile of isoflavone intake (Hazard ratio=0.66, 95% CI, p=0.01) (Kang *et al*, 2010, p.1859). Specifically, the recurrence rate among women in the highest quartile was 12% lower than recurrence rates in the lowest quartile. This study therefore shows that isoflavone consumption can reduce breast cancer risks in women.

On the other hand, some studies have shown that isoflavones can cause breast cancer. A clinical study published in the *Nutritional Journal* by Messina and Wood (2008, p.6) has shown that isoflavones are a possible risk factor for breast cancer among women. In this study, breast nipple aspirate (NAF) was collected from 37 women participants (Messina & Wood, 2008, p.6). These samples were collected for three months before the participants were exposed to isoflavone consumption. Samples were also collected during six months of isoflavone consumption and three months after discontinuation of exposure to isoflavone (Messina & Wood, 2008, p.6).

Participants were provided with 75mg of isoflavones each day during the six months of exposure. After analysis, it was found that 29% of the participants had experienced increased levels of breast cancer cell growth (Messina & Wood, 2008, p.6). Consequently, the participants reported increase in tumor sizes, an incident that could only mean that isoflavones were indeed enhancing the growth of cancerous cells in the mammary tissues of the victims (Messina & Wood, 2008, p.6). However, this study had the limitation of being a pilot project; hence no concrete conclusions can be made based on the study.

Conclusion

Isoflavones in soy foods have been found to inhibit breast cancer in women. Despite the controversy that surrounds the effects of isoflavones on this disease, mitigation characteristics of isoflavones against breast cancer outweigh the limitations. Thus, it is prudent to say that consumption of isoflavones is helpful in the treatment or prevention of breast cancer. Isoflavones are capable of causing various biological actions to take place. Such actions which inhibit growth of cancerous cells include slowed epidermal development of tyrosine kinase, inhibited angiogenesis and modification of eicosanoid metabolism. However, these anticancer effects occur when isoflavone compounds are consumed at pharmacologic concentrations. Isoflavones are beneficial in reducing cancer recurrence rates in women. As such, the strong points of isoflavone consumption surpass the risks, and it can be concluded that soy foods inhibit breast cancer. Thus, the hypothesis investigated in this research is true, since there is a stronger argument for including soy foods in the female diet.

8

References

Kang, X. *et al*, (2010). Effect of soy isoflavones on breast cancer recurrence and death for patients receiving adjuvant endocrine therapy. *Canadian medical association*, 182(17), 1857-1862.

Messina, M. & Wu, A. H. (2009). Perspectives on the soy-breast cancer relation. *American journal of clinical nutrition, 89*, 1673-1679.

Messina, M. J., & Wood, C. E. (2008). Soy isoflavones, estrogen therapy and breast cancer risk: analysis and commentary. *Nutrition journal, 7*(17), 1-11.

Nagata, C. (2010). Factors to consider in the association between soy isoflavone intake and breast cancer risk. *Journal of epidemiology, 20*(2), 83-89.

Trock, B. J., Hilakivi-Clarke, L., & Clarke, R. (2006). Meta-analysis of soy intake and breast cancer risk. *Journal of the National Cancer Institute, 98*(7), 459-471.

Wu, A. H. *et al*, (2008). Soy intake and breast cancer risk in Singapore Chinese health study. *British journal of cancer, 99*(1), 196-200.